I0841686

Published by Fitness Marketing Group, Sunrise Beach, MO

Printed in the United States of America.

ISBN: 9798856549385

This publication is designed to provide accurate and authoritative information with regard to the subject matter covered. It is sold with the understanding that the publisher is not engaged in rendering legal, accounting, or other professional advice. If expert or professional assistance is required, the services of a competent professional should be sought.

First edition

For more information, contact:

JayLab Pro, Inc
2025 Zumbehl Road PMB13
Saint Charles, MO 63301
1 (888) 943-8776

Visit us online at: www.JayLabPro.com

Chapter 1: Understanding the Liver's Vital Role in Health
- *The liver's functions and its significance in overall well-being*
- *Exploring the impact of liver health on various bodily systems*

Chapter 2: Uncovering the Signs of Liver Dysfunction
- *Recognizing common symptoms and indicators of liver problems*
- *Understanding the importance of early detection and intervention*

Chapter 3: Nourishing Your Liver: The Power of a Healthy Diet
- *Exploring liver-friendly foods and their impact on rejuvenation*
- *Creating a balanced and nutritious meal plan to support liver health*

Chapter 4: Detoxification Strategies for Liver Rejuvenation
- *Understanding the liver's role in detoxification*
- *Implementing effective detox methods to support liver function*

Chapter 5: Herbs and Supplements for Liver Rejuvenation
- *Exploring natural remedies that promote liver health*
- *Understanding the benefits and proper usage of liver-supportive herbs and supplements*

Chapter 6: Lifestyle Habits for a Healthy Liver
- *The impact of alcohol, smoking, and stress on liver function*
- *Adopting lifestyle changes to support liver rejuvenation*

Chapter 7: Exercise for Liver Health and Rejuvenation
- *Unveiling the relationship between physical activity and liver function*
- *Designing an exercise routine that benefits liver health*

Chapter 8: Sleep and Liver Rejuvenation
- *The importance of quality sleep in liver rejuvenation*
- *Tips for improving sleep habits to support liver health*

Chapter 9: Mind-Body Connection: Mental Wellness for Liver Rejuvenation
- *Exploring the link between emotional well-being and liver health*
- *Strategies for managing stress, anxiety, and promoting mental wellness*

Chapter 10: Long-Term Liver Rejuvenation: Maintenance and Prevention
- *Maintaining a healthy liver beyond rejuvenation*
- *Preventive measures to ensure long-term liver health and vitality*

Introduction: The Liver Rejuvenation Blueprint: Unlocking Your Body's Vitality

Welcome to "The Liver Rejuvenation Blueprint: Unlocking Your Body's Vitality." In this comprehensive guide, we will embark on a transformative journey to understand and optimize the health of one of the most crucial organs in our body—the liver. By delving into the intricacies of liver rejuvenation, we will unlock the key to unlocking our body's vitality and achieving optimal well-being.

The liver, often referred to as the body's powerhouse, is a remarkable organ that performs an array of vital functions necessary for our overall health. It is responsible for detoxifying harmful substances, synthesizing essential proteins, regulating metabolism, storing nutrients, aiding in digestion, and maintaining immune function. A healthy liver is essential for our physical, mental, and emotional well-being.

However, in today's modern world, our liver faces numerous challenges. Poor dietary choices, sedentary lifestyles, exposure to environmental toxins, excessive alcohol consumption, and chronic stress can take a toll on the health of our liver. Over time, these factors can lead to liver dysfunction, inflammation, and the development of various liver-related diseases.

But here's the good news: our liver possesses an incredible ability to regenerate and rejuvenate itself. With the right knowledge, strategies, and commitment, we can restore and optimize the health of our liver, allowing it to function at its full potential. This is where "The Liver Rejuvenation Blueprint" comes into play.

In this book, we will guide you through a comprehensive roadmap for liver rejuvenation, empowering you to take charge of your liver health and unlock your body's vitality. We will explore the critical aspects of liver rejuvenation, including understanding the liver's vital role in health, uncovering the signs of liver dysfunction, nourishing your liver with a healthy diet, implementing effective detoxification strategies, harnessing the power of herbs and supplements, adopting lifestyle habits for a healthy liver, utilizing exercise for liver health, optimizing sleep, fostering mental wellness, and establishing long-term maintenance and preventive measures.

Each chapter is designed to provide you with valuable insights, practical tips, and evidence-based strategies that you can incorporate into your daily life. We will unravel the interconnectedness of the liver with various bodily systems, helping you understand how liver health influences overall well-being. From dietary recommendations to stress management techniques, we will equip you with the tools to make informed decisions and take proactive steps towards liver rejuvenation.

It is important to note that this book is not intended as a substitute for professional medical advice. If you have pre-existing liver conditions or any concerns about your liver health, we encourage you to consult with a healthcare professional for personalized guidance and support.

Are you ready to embark on this transformative journey? Are you ready to unlock the vitality and well-being that your body deserves? "The Liver Rejuvenation Blueprint" is your comprehensive guide to revitalizing your liver and reclaiming your health. Let's dive in and unlock the incredible potential of your body's powerhouse—the liver.

Chapter 1: Understanding the Liver's Vital Role in Health

The liver is a remarkable organ that plays a crucial role in maintaining our overall health and well-being. It performs numerous functions essential for the proper functioning of our body systems, and any disruption in its health can have significant consequences. In this chapter, we will delve into the functions of the liver and explore the impact of liver health on various bodily systems.

The Functions of the Liver:

The liver is the largest internal organ in the human body, located in the upper right quadrant of the abdomen. It is involved in a wide range of metabolic, digestive, and detoxification processes. Let's explore some of the key functions of the liver:

1. Metabolism: The liver plays a central role in metabolic processes. It regulates the storage and release of glucose, ensuring a steady supply of energy for the body. It also metabolizes fats, converting them into energy and producing cholesterol for hormone synthesis.

2. Detoxification: One of the liver's primary functions is to detoxify harmful substances in the body. It filters and removes toxins, drugs, and metabolic waste products, preventing them from circulating in the bloodstream. The liver breaks down these substances

into less harmful forms that can be eliminated through bile or urine.

3. Protein Synthesis: The liver synthesizes proteins essential for various bodily functions. It produces albumin, a protein that helps maintain osmotic pressure in blood vessels, and clotting factors that are crucial for blood coagulation. Additionally, the liver synthesizes proteins involved in immune function and hormone regulation.

4. Bile Production: The liver produces bile, a greenish-yellow fluid necessary for the digestion and absorption of fats. Bile is stored in the gallbladder and released into the small intestine when fat is consumed. It aids in the emulsification and breakdown of dietary fats, enabling their absorption into the bloodstream.

5. Nutrient Storage: The liver acts as a storage site for several essential nutrients. It stores glycogen, a complex carbohydrate that can be broken down into glucose when the body needs an immediate energy supply. The liver also stores vitamins (A, D, E, K, and B12), minerals (iron and copper), and fatty acids.

The Impact of Liver Health on Various Bodily Systems:

The health of the liver has a profound impact on the functioning of various bodily systems. Let's explore some of these systems and the consequences of liver dysfunction:

1. Digestive System: The liver plays a crucial role in the digestion and metabolism of nutrients. Liver dysfunction can impair bile production and disrupt the digestion and absorption of fats, leading to nutrient deficiencies and malabsorption. It can also result in conditions such as jaundice, where bilirubin, a yellow pigment produced during the breakdown of red blood cells, accumulates in the body.

2. Metabolic System: The liver regulates glucose metabolism, helping to maintain stable blood sugar levels. Dysfunction of the liver can lead to glucose dysregulation, resulting in conditions such as insulin resistance and diabetes. It can also contribute to the accumulation of triglycerides and cholesterol in the bloodstream, increasing the risk of cardiovascular diseases.

3. Immune System: The liver plays a vital role in immune function. It helps remove bacteria, viruses, and other pathogens from the bloodstream, preventing their spread throughout the body. Liver dysfunction can weaken the immune system, making individuals more susceptible to infections and impairing the body's ability to fight off diseases.

4. Detoxification System: The liver is the primary organ responsible for detoxifying harmful substances. When the liver is compromised, toxins can build up in the body, causing oxidative stress and damage to cells and tissues. This can lead to various health issues, including liver diseases, metabolic disorders, and an increased risk of developing chronic conditions such as liver cirrhosis and liver cancer.

5. Cardiovascular System: Liver health is closely linked to cardiovascular health. The liver produces proteins involved in blood clotting, and dysfunction of the liver can disrupt the clotting process, leading to an increased risk of bleeding disorders or thrombosis. Additionally, liver dysfunction can contribute to the accumulation of cholesterol and triglycerides in the blood, promoting the development of atherosclerosis and cardiovascular diseases.

6. Hormonal Regulation: The liver plays a significant role in hormone regulation. It metabolizes hormones such as estrogen, testosterone, and thyroid hormones, ensuring their proper balance in the body. Liver dysfunction can disrupt hormone metabolism, leading to hormonal imbalances, reproductive issues, and other endocrine disorders.

7. Central Nervous System: Liver health has an impact on the central nervous system. The liver metabolizes ammonia, a toxic substance produced during protein metabolism, into urea, which is then eliminated through urine. When the liver is not functioning optimally, ammonia can accumulate in the bloodstream, leading to a condition known as hepatic encephalopathy. This condition can cause neurological symptoms such as confusion, cognitive impairment, and even coma.

Conclusion:
The liver's vital role in maintaining overall health and well-being cannot be overstated. Its functions encompass metabolism, detoxification, digestion, and immune support, among others. A healthy liver is essential for the proper functioning of various bodily systems, including the digestive, metabolic, immune, cardiovascular, and hormonal systems.

Understanding the significance of liver health empowers us to prioritize its well-being. By adopting a healthy lifestyle, including a balanced diet, regular exercise, moderate alcohol consumption, and avoiding hepatotoxic substances, we can support liver health and prevent liver dysfunction. Regular check-ups, early detection, and prompt intervention are crucial in managing liver conditions and preserving liver function.

In the following chapters, we will explore various aspects of liver rejuvenation, including diet, exercise, detoxification, and lifestyle habits that can promote liver health and vitality. By implementing these strategies, we can optimize liver function, enhance overall well-being, and reduce the risk of liver-related diseases.

Chapter 2: Uncovering the Signs of Liver Dysfunction

Recognizing common symptoms and indicators of liver problems

Understanding the importance of early detection and intervention

Introduction:
The liver, being a vital organ responsible for numerous essential functions in the body, can sometimes experience dysfunction or damage. It is crucial to recognize the signs and symptoms of liver problems at an early stage to facilitate timely intervention and prevent the progression of liver diseases. In this chapter, we will explore the common indicators of liver dysfunction and emphasize the significance of early detection and intervention.

The Silent Nature of Liver Disorders:

Liver disorders often exhibit subtle symptoms in their early stages, making them challenging to identify. The liver possesses remarkable regenerative capabilities, allowing it to compensate for minor damage without manifesting apparent signs. Unfortunately, this silent nature can lead to undiagnosed liver problems, which may progress into more severe conditions if left untreated.

Common Signs and Symptoms of Liver Dysfunction:

While liver diseases may initially be asymptomatic, there are several indicators that can suggest the presence of liver dysfunction. It is important to note that experiencing one or more of these signs does not necessarily mean liver disease, but they serve as potential warning signs that warrant further investigation. Some common signs and symptoms include:

Jaundice:

Jaundice is characterized by the yellowing of the skin, eyes, and mucous membranes. It occurs when bilirubin, a yellow pigment produced during the breakdown of red blood cells, accumulates in the body due to impaired liver function. Jaundice can indicate various liver disorders, such as hepatitis, cirrhosis, or liver cancer.

Fatigue and Weakness:

Persistent fatigue and weakness are frequently associated with liver dysfunction. The liver plays a vital role in energy metabolism and nutrient storage. When it is compromised, energy levels may decline, leading to fatigue, weakness, and a general sense of lethargy.

Abdominal Pain and Swelling:

Liver disorders can cause abdominal discomfort or pain. The liver itself does not have pain receptors, but inflammation or enlargement of the liver can cause stretching of the liver capsule, resulting in pain or a feeling of fullness in the upper right abdomen. Additionally, fluid accumulation in the abdominal cavity, known as ascites, may cause abdominal swelling.

Digestive Issues:

Liver dysfunction can disrupt the digestive process, leading to various gastrointestinal symptoms. These may include loss of appetite, nausea, vomiting, diarrhea, or changes in bowel movements. Fat malabsorption and deficiency of bile, which aids in fat digestion, can result in greasy stools or pale-colored stools.

Dark Urine and Pale Stools:

Liver problems can alter the color of urine and stools. Dark urine, often resembling the color of cola, occurs due to the presence of bilirubin. Conversely, stools may appear pale or clay-colored due to insufficient bile reaching the intestines.

Unexplained Weight Loss or Gain:

Liver dysfunction can disrupt the metabolism of nutrients, leading to unexplained weight loss or weight gain. In some cases, liver diseases may cause a loss of appetite, resulting in unintentional weight loss. Conversely, fluid retention or fat accumulation can contribute to unexplained weight gain.

Importance of Early Detection and Intervention:

Early detection and intervention play a crucial role in managing liver disorders effectively. By identifying liver dysfunction in its initial stages, medical professionals can implement appropriate treatments and lifestyle modifications to prevent further damage and potentially reverse the condition. Here are some reasons why early detection is essential:

Preventing Disease Progression:

Liver diseases, if left untreated, can progress and lead to irreversible damage such as cirrhosis or liver cancer. Early detection allows for timely intervention, which can slow down or halt the progression of the disease. By addressing liver dysfunction in its early stages, the chances of successful treatment and management are significantly improved.

Promoting Better Treatment Outcomes:

Early detection enables healthcare professionals to implement appropriate treatment strategies promptly. This may include lifestyle modifications, medications, or interventions tailored to the specific liver condition. When liver diseases are identified early, there is a higher likelihood of achieving positive treatment outcomes and preserving liver function.

Managing Underlying Causes:

Liver dysfunction can stem from various underlying causes, including viral infections (such as hepatitis B or C), excessive alcohol consumption, fatty liver disease, autoimmune disorders, or certain medications. Early detection allows for a thorough evaluation of the potential causes, which can guide targeted treatments or lifestyle adjustments. By addressing the root cause, it becomes possible to manage liver dysfunction more effectively.

Reducing Complications:

Liver disorders can lead to complications that can significantly impact overall health. For instance, advanced liver disease can result in portal hypertension, the development of varices (enlarged blood vessels) in the esophagus or stomach, and an increased risk of bleeding. Early detection and intervention can help prevent or manage these complications, reducing the risk of severe consequences.

Improving Quality of Life:

Liver dysfunction can have a profound impact on an individual's quality of life. Symptoms such as fatigue, abdominal pain, and digestive issues can significantly impair daily activities and overall well-being. Early detection and appropriate management can alleviate these symptoms, improve energy levels, and enhance overall quality of life.

Empowering Lifestyle Changes:

Early detection of liver dysfunction provides an opportunity for individuals to make necessary lifestyle changes. By addressing risk factors such as excessive alcohol consumption, unhealthy diet, obesity, or certain medications, individuals can actively participate in their liver health management and make informed choices that support liver rejuvenation.

Conclusion:

Recognizing the signs and symptoms of liver dysfunction and understanding the importance of early detection and intervention are crucial steps in maintaining liver health. By being aware of common indicators such as jaundice, fatigue, abdominal pain, and digestive issues, individuals can seek medical attention promptly, leading to timely diagnosis and appropriate management. Early detection not only prevents disease progression but also improves treatment outcomes, reduces complications, and enhances quality of life. Prioritizing liver health through regular check-ups, healthy lifestyle choices, and awareness empowers individuals to take proactive measures in unlocking their body's vitality and ensuring long-term well-being.

Chapter 3: Nourishing Your Liver: The Power of a Healthy Diet

Exploring liver-friendly foods and their impact on rejuvenation

Creating a balanced and nutritious meal plan to support liver health

Introduction:
The food we consume plays a critical role in supporting liver health and rejuvenation. A healthy diet not only provides essential nutrients but also helps optimize liver function and promote overall well-being. In this chapter, we will explore liver-friendly foods and their impact on liver rejuvenation. Additionally, we will discuss strategies for creating a balanced and nutritious meal plan to support optimal liver health.

Understanding Liver-Friendly Foods:

Liver-friendly foods are those that provide essential nutrients, antioxidants, and compounds that support liver function, aid in detoxification, and reduce inflammation. These foods help nourish and rejuvenate the liver, allowing it to perform its vital tasks efficiently. Here are some liver-friendly foods to incorporate into your diet:

Cruciferous Vegetables:

Cruciferous vegetables such as broccoli, cauliflower, cabbage, and Brussels sprouts contain compounds like glucosinolates, which support liver detoxification processes. They also provide important antioxidants and fiber, promoting overall digestive health.

Leafy Greens:

Leafy greens like spinach, kale, and Swiss chard are rich in vitamins, minerals, and antioxidants that help protect the liver from oxidative stress. They also contain chlorophyll, which aids in detoxification.

Berries:

Berries, such as blueberries, strawberries, and raspberries, are packed with antioxidants that help reduce inflammation and protect liver cells from damage. They are also high in fiber, which supports healthy digestion.

Citrus Fruits:

Citrus fruits like oranges, lemons, and grapefruits are excellent sources of vitamin C, a potent antioxidant that helps boost the immune system and supports liver detoxification processes.

Garlic and Onions:

Garlic and onions contain sulfur compounds that support the liver's natural detoxification pathways. They also possess anti-inflammatory properties and may help reduce liver inflammation.

Turmeric:

Turmeric contains a powerful compound called curcumin, known for its antioxidant and anti-inflammatory properties. Curcumin helps protect liver cells and supports liver regeneration.

A great source is Fermented Turmeric. Learn more about Fermented Turmeric here: **www.jaylabpro.com/fermented-turmeric.html**

Walnuts:

Walnuts are a good source of healthy fats, including omega-3 fatty acids and antioxidants. They also contain arginine, an amino acid that aids in liver detoxification processes.

Green Tea:

Green tea is rich in catechins, a type of antioxidant that has been shown to protect liver cells from damage and promote liver health.

Designing a Liver-Friendly Meal Plan:

To create a balanced and nutritious meal plan that supports liver health, consider the following guidelines:

See Appendix A at the end of this book.

Prioritize Whole Foods:

Focus on consuming whole, unprocessed foods that provide a wide range of nutrients. Include plenty of fresh fruits, vegetables, whole grains, lean proteins, and healthy fats in your diet.

Include Lean Proteins:

Incorporate lean protein sources such as fish, poultry, legumes, and tofu into your meals. These provide essential amino acids for liver cell regeneration and repair.

Opt for Healthy Fats:

Include healthy fats from sources like avocados, olive oil, nuts, and seeds. These fats provide essential fatty acids that support liver health and help reduce inflammation.

Emphasize Fiber-Rich Foods:

Include high-fiber foods such as whole grains, legumes, fruits, and vegetables in your meals. Fiber aids in digestion, promotes regular bowel movements, and supports the elimination of toxins from the body.

Limit Processed and Sugary Foods:

Reduce or avoid processed foods, refined sugars, and artificial additives, as they can burden the liver and contribute to inflammation. Opt for natural sweeteners like honey or maple syrup when needed.

Stay Hydrated:

Proper hydration is essential for liver function and overall health. Aim to drink an adequate amount of water throughout the day to support detoxification processes and maintain optimal liver function.

Moderate Alcohol Consumption:

Excessive alcohol consumption can cause liver damage. If you choose to drink alcohol, do so in moderation and be mindful of your limits. For those with liver conditions or seeking optimal liver health, it is best to avoid alcohol altogether.

Consider Portion Sizes:

Maintain portion control and listen to your body's hunger and fullness cues. Overeating can strain the liver and contribute to weight gain, while consistently eating smaller, balanced meals supports digestion and overall liver health.

Creating Liver-Friendly Meal Ideas:

To help you get started, here are a few liver-friendly meal ideas that incorporate the aforementioned foods:

- Grilled salmon with steamed broccoli and quinoa
- Spinach and kale salad with citrus fruits, walnuts, and a lemon-turmeric dressing
- Stir-fried tofu with mixed vegetables, garlic, and ginger
- Whole grain wrap filled with grilled chicken, leafy greens, and sliced onions
- Quinoa and vegetable stir-fry with added cruciferous vegetables and a splash of soy sauce
- Overnight chia seed pudding made with almond milk, topped with berries and a sprinkle of ground flaxseeds
- Green tea-infused smoothie bowl with spinach, banana, avocado, and a sprinkle of nuts or seeds for added crunch

Remember, these are just a few examples, and you can mix and match ingredients to create your own liver-friendly meals. Be creative, experiment with flavors, and enjoy the process of nourishing your liver through delicious and nutritious food.

In Appendix B I share multiple liver detoxification recipes.

Conclusion:

A healthy diet plays a vital role in supporting liver health and rejuvenation. By incorporating liver-friendly foods such as cruciferous vegetables, leafy greens, berries, citrus fruits, garlic, onions, turmeric, walnuts, and green tea into your meals, you can provide essential nutrients, antioxidants, and compounds that support optimal liver function.

Designing a balanced and nutritious meal plan that prioritizes whole foods, lean proteins, healthy fats, fiber, hydration, and portion control further enhances liver health.

By embracing a liver-friendly diet, you empower yourself to take an active role in unlocking your body's vitality and promoting long-term well-being.

Remember, small dietary changes can make a significant impact on liver health, so start nourishing your liver today and reap the benefits of a healthier, rejuvenated you.

Special Report:

At the link below I have a special report for you to download called ***"14 Foods That Heal Your Liver (and also ignite your Fat Burning Hormones)"***.

It is a great addition to this book and helps with rejuvenating your liver.

Grab the report here:
www. jaylabpro.com/14-Foods-Heal-Liver.html

Chapter 4: Detoxification Strategies for Liver Rejuvenation

Understanding the liver's role in detoxification

Implementing effective detox methods to support liver function

Introduction:

The liver is the body's primary detoxification organ, responsible for filtering toxins, waste products, and harmful substances from the bloodstream. However, in today's world, our bodies are exposed to an increasing number of toxins from various sources, including pollution, processed foods, and chemicals. This puts a strain on the liver and can lead to impaired detoxification function. In this chapter, we will explore the liver's role in detoxification, understand the importance of supporting its function, and discuss effective detox strategies to promote liver rejuvenation.

The Liver's Role in Detoxification:

The liver performs a complex series of biochemical reactions to neutralize and eliminate toxins from the body. It transforms harmful substances into less harmful or water-soluble forms that can be excreted through urine or bile. Here are the primary mechanisms by which the liver detoxifies:

Phase I Detoxification:

In Phase I, the liver enzymes convert fat-soluble toxins into intermediate metabolites. This process involves various reactions, including oxidation, reduction, and hydrolysis, to make the toxins more accessible for further processing.

Phase II Detoxification:

In Phase II, the intermediate metabolites from Phase I are conjugated with other substances, such as amino acids, sulfur, or glucuronic acid, to form water-soluble compounds. These water-soluble compounds are easier to eliminate from the body through urine or bile.

Bile Production and Excretion:

The liver produces bile, a substance that helps emulsify fats and carries waste products, toxins, and cholesterol out of the liver. Bile is then excreted into the small intestine, where it aids in the digestion and elimination of these substances.

Supporting Liver Detoxification:

To support liver function and enhance the detoxification process, it is essential to adopt healthy lifestyle practices and implement effective detox strategies. Here are some approaches to consider:

Nutrient-Rich Diet:

Eating a nutrient-dense diet provides the liver with the necessary vitamins, minerals, and antioxidants it needs for optimal detoxification. Include foods rich in antioxidants, such as colorful fruits and vegetables, as well as sulfur-containing foods like garlic, onions, and cruciferous vegetables. Additionally, ensure an adequate intake of vitamins B, C, and E, as well as minerals like selenium and zinc.

Hydration:

Proper hydration is crucial for supporting liver detoxification. Drinking an adequate amount of water helps flush out toxins and ensures optimal liver function. Aim to consume at least 8 glasses of water per day and consider incorporating herbal teas or infused water for added benefits.

Regular Exercise:

Engaging in regular physical activity promotes blood circulation, lymphatic flow, and sweating, which aids in toxin elimination. Exercise also helps maintain a healthy weight, reduces inflammation, and supports overall liver health. Aim for at least 30 minutes of moderate-intensity exercise most days of the week.

Minimize Exposure to Toxins:

Reducing your exposure to toxins can lessen the burden on the liver. Avoid or minimize contact with environmental toxins, such as air pollution, pesticides, and harsh cleaning chemicals. Choose natural and organic personal care and household products whenever possible.

Sleep and Stress Management:

Adequate sleep and effective stress management are essential for liver health. Poor sleep and chronic stress can impair liver function and hinder the detoxification process. Prioritize quality sleep and adopt stress-reducing practices, such as meditation, deep breathing exercises, yoga, or engaging in activities that bring you joy and relaxation.

Liver-Supportive Supplements:

Certain supplements can assist in liver detoxification. Milk thistle, a well-known herb, contains a compound called silymarin that has been shown to protect liver cells and support their regeneration. Other supplements, such as turmeric, dandelion root, and N-acetyl cysteine (NAC), also have liver-supportive properties. However, it is important to consult with a healthcare professional before starting any new supplements to ensure they are appropriate for your specific needs.

Sauna Therapy:

Sauna therapy is a method that utilizes heat to induce sweating and facilitate toxin elimination through the skin. Regular sauna sessions can support the liver's detoxification efforts and promote overall well-being. However, it is important to stay properly hydrated during and after sauna sessions to avoid dehydration.

Intermittent Fasting:

Intermittent fasting is an eating pattern that involves cycling between periods of fasting and eating. This approach can support liver detoxification by giving the liver a break from constant digestion and allowing it to focus on detoxification processes. Consult with a healthcare professional before incorporating intermittent fasting into your routine, especially if you have any underlying health conditions.

Conclusion:

Supporting the liver's detoxification function is crucial for maintaining overall health and promoting liver rejuvenation. By understanding the liver's role in detoxification and implementing effective strategies such as following a nutrient-rich diet, staying hydrated, exercising regularly, minimizing toxin exposure, managing stress, considering liver-supportive supplements, exploring sauna therapy, and incorporating intermittent fasting, you can optimize your liver's ability to eliminate toxins and promote its rejuvenation. Remember to personalize your detoxification plan to suit your specific needs and consult with a healthcare professional before making any significant changes. By prioritizing liver detoxification, you unlock the potential for improved health, increased vitality, and a stronger foundation for overall well-being.

To accelerate your detoxification efforts you can incorporate a cleanse supplement that contains some of the nutrients mentioned in the chapter below as well as other liver detoxifying nutrients.

Here is a great liver detoxifying supplement you can add to your liver rejuvenation process.

https://www.jaylabpro.com/ultra-cleanse.html

Chapter 5: Herbs and Supplements for Liver Rejuvenation

Exploring natural remedies that promote liver health

Understanding the benefits and proper usage of liver-supportive herbs and supplements

Introduction:

In addition to adopting a healthy diet and lifestyle, incorporating herbs and supplements into your routine can provide valuable support for liver rejuvenation. Certain herbs and supplements have been traditionally used for centuries due to their liver-protective and detoxifying properties. In this chapter, we will explore various natural remedies that promote liver health, understand their benefits, and discuss the proper usage of liver-supportive herbs and supplements.

Milk Thistle (Silybum marianum):

Milk thistle is one of the most well-known herbs for liver health. It contains a compound called silymarin, which has potent antioxidant and anti-inflammatory properties. Silymarin helps protect liver cells from damage, supports liver regeneration, and aids in detoxification processes. Milk thistle is commonly available as a standardized extract in capsule or liquid form. The typical recommended dosage is 200-400 mg of silymarin per day. It is advisable to consult with a healthcare professional before starting milk thistle or any new supplement.

Dandelion Root (Taraxacum officinale):

Dandelion root has a long history of traditional use in promoting liver health. It supports liver detoxification by stimulating bile production and improving liver function. Dandelion root is available as a tea, tincture, or capsule. Drinking dandelion root tea or taking a dandelion root supplement can help support liver health. Follow the recommended dosage on the product label or consult with a healthcare professional for guidance.

Turmeric (Curcuma longa):

Turmeric is a vibrant yellow spice widely used in cooking and traditional medicine. It contains an active compound called curcumin, which has potent anti-inflammatory and antioxidant properties. Curcumin supports liver health by reducing inflammation, protecting liver cells, and promoting liver regeneration. Turmeric can be added to your diet as a spice or taken in supplement form. The recommended dosage for turmeric supplements typically ranges from 500-2,000 mg per day, standardized to contain a specific percentage of curcumin. Consult with a healthcare professional for personalized dosage recommendations.

Artichoke Leaf (Cynara scolymus):

Artichoke leaf has been traditionally used to support liver health and digestion. It contains compounds that stimulate bile production, enhance liver function, and aid in detoxification. Artichoke leaf extract is available in capsule or tincture form. The recommended dosage varies, but a typical range is 300-600 mg of artichoke leaf extract per day. It is advisable to consult with a healthcare professional for personalized dosage recommendations.

Schisandra (Schisandra chinensis):

Schisandra is an adaptogenic herb used in traditional Chinese medicine to support liver health and overall vitality. It helps protect the liver from toxins, reduce inflammation, and enhance liver function. Schisandra is available as a supplement in capsule or liquid extract form. The recommended dosage varies, but a typical range is 500-1,500 mg per day. Consult with a healthcare professional for personalized dosage recommendations.

N-Acetyl Cysteine (NAC):

N-Acetyl Cysteine (NAC) is a powerful antioxidant that supports liver health. It helps replenish glutathione, a key antioxidant produced by the liver, which plays a crucial role in detoxification processes. NAC is available in capsule or powder form. The recommended dosage typically ranges from 600-1,800 mg per day. However, it is important to consult with a healthcare professional, as NAC may interact with certain medications or health conditions.

Burdock Root (Arctium lappa):

Burdock root is a herb commonly used in traditional herbal medicine for liver support. It helps enhance liver function, promote detoxification, and reduce inflammation. Burdock root is available in various forms, including capsules, tinctures, or dried root for tea. The recommended dosage varies, but a typical range is 1-2 grams of dried root or 2-6 mL of tincture per day. Consult with a healthcare professional for personalized dosage recommendations.

Alpha-Lipoic Acid (ALA):

Alpha-Lipoic Acid (ALA) is a powerful antioxidant that supports liver health and helps regenerate other antioxidants, such as glutathione and vitamins C and E. It also helps protect liver cells from oxidative damage. ALA is available in capsule or tablet form. The recommended dosage varies, but a typical range is 300-600 mg per day. Consult with a healthcare professional for personalized dosage recommendations.

Globe Artichoke (Cynara cardunculus):

Globe artichoke is another herb with liver-protective properties. It supports liver function, promotes bile production, and aids in detoxification processes. Globe artichoke is available in various forms, including capsules, extracts, or as part of a liver support blend. The recommended dosage varies, but a typical range is 300-640 mg of standardized extract per day. Consult with a healthcare professional for personalized dosage recommendations.

Green Tea (Camellia sinensis):

Green tea is known for its high content of antioxidants, including catechins. These compounds help reduce liver inflammation, protect liver cells, and support liver function. Regular consumption of green tea can contribute to overall liver health. Aim to drink 2-3 cups of green tea per day to harness its benefits.

Conclusion:

Incorporating liver-supportive herbs and supplements into your routine can be a valuable addition to a healthy lifestyle and diet for liver rejuvenation. Milk thistle, dandelion root, turmeric, artichoke leaf, schisandra, N-acetyl cysteine (NAC), burdock root, alpha-lipoic acid (ALA), globe artichoke, and green tea are among the herbs and supplements known for their liver-protective and detoxifying properties.

When using herbs and supplements, it is important to follow recommended dosages, consult with a healthcare professional if you have any underlying health conditions or are taking medications, and ensure the quality and safety of the products you choose. While these natural remedies can support liver health, they are not a substitute for medical treatment or a healthy lifestyle. Remember to prioritize a balanced diet, regular exercise, adequate hydration, and stress management for comprehensive liver rejuvenation.

By harnessing the power of nature's remedies and supporting your liver through the use of herbs and supplements, you can unlock your body's innate ability to detoxify, regenerate, and promote optimal liver health. Embrace these natural tools as part of your liver rejuvenation journey and experience the benefits of a revitalized and healthier you.

Chapter 6: Lifestyle Habits for a Healthy Liver

The impact of alcohol, smoking, and stress on liver function

Adopting lifestyle changes to support liver rejuvenation

Introduction:

The liver plays a vital role in our overall health and well-being. It is responsible for detoxifying harmful substances, metabolizing nutrients, producing bile for digestion, and storing essential vitamins and minerals. However, certain lifestyle habits can have a significant impact on liver function. In this chapter, we will explore the effects of alcohol, smoking, and stress on the liver, as well as discuss lifestyle changes that can support liver rejuvenation.

The Impact of Alcohol on Liver Function:

Excessive alcohol consumption can have a detrimental effect on the liver. Alcohol is processed by the liver, and chronic alcohol abuse can lead to various liver conditions, including fatty liver disease, alcoholic hepatitis, and cirrhosis. These conditions can impair liver function, disrupt the liver's ability to detoxify the body, and increase the risk of liver damage.

To support liver health, it is crucial to adopt moderate alcohol consumption or, ideally, abstain from alcohol altogether. For men, moderate alcohol consumption is defined as up to two standard drinks per day, while for women, it is up to one standard drink per day. It is important to note that these guidelines may vary depending on individual circumstances, and individuals with existing liver conditions or health concerns should avoid alcohol completely. If you are struggling with alcohol consumption, seeking professional help and support is essential.

The Impact of Smoking on Liver Function:

Smoking cigarettes not only affects the lungs but also has a negative impact on liver health. The toxins in cigarette smoke are absorbed into the bloodstream and processed by the liver. Prolonged smoking can lead to the accumulation of harmful substances in the liver, causing inflammation and damage to liver cells.

Quitting smoking is crucial for liver rejuvenation and overall health. By quitting smoking, you can reduce the risk of developing liver diseases and improve liver function. There are various methods and resources available to help individuals quit smoking, including nicotine replacement therapy, counseling, support groups, and medications. It may take time and perseverance, but the benefits to your liver and overall well-being are well worth it.

The Impact of Stress on Liver Function:

Chronic stress can have a significant impact on liver health. When we experience stress, the body releases stress hormones such as cortisol, which, when elevated over a prolonged period, can lead to inflammation and damage to the liver. Stress can also contribute to unhealthy coping mechanisms, such as excessive alcohol consumption or poor dietary choices, further burdening the liver.

To support liver rejuvenation, it is crucial to manage stress effectively. Adopting stress management techniques such as meditation, deep breathing exercises, yoga, mindfulness practices, and engaging in activities that bring joy and relaxation can help reduce stress levels. Regular exercise, quality sleep, and maintaining a healthy work-life balance are also important factors in managing stress and supporting liver health.

Lifestyle Changes for Liver Rejuvenation:

In addition to avoiding alcohol, quitting smoking, and managing stress, there are several lifestyle changes you can make to support liver rejuvenation:

Follow a Balanced and Nutritious Diet:

A diet rich in fruits, vegetables, whole grains, lean proteins, and healthy fats provides essential nutrients for liver health. Avoid or minimize processed foods, sugary snacks, and excessive consumption of saturated and trans fats, as these can contribute to liver damage and inflammation. Incorporate liver-friendly foods such as leafy greens, cruciferous vegetables, garlic, onions, berries, citrus fruits, turmeric, and green tea.

Maintain a Healthy Weight:

Obesity and excess body weight can increase the risk of fatty liver disease and other liver conditions. By adopting a healthy lifestyle that includes regular exercise and a balanced diet, you can achieve and maintain a healthy weight, reducing the strain on your liver and promoting its rejuvenation.

Stay Hydrated:

Adequate hydration is essential for liver health. Water helps flush out toxins and waste products from the body, supporting the liver's detoxification processes. Aim to drink an adequate amount of water throughout the day and limit your intake of sugary beverages and alcohol, as they can further burden the liver.

Exercise Regularly:

Regular physical activity has numerous benefits for liver health. Exercise helps improve blood circulation, which aids in the delivery of nutrients to the liver and the removal of toxins. Engage in activities that you enjoy, such as walking, jogging, cycling, swimming, or participating in sports. Aim for at least 30 minutes of moderate-intensity exercise most days of the week.

Get Sufficient Sleep:

Quality sleep is crucial for liver rejuvenation. During sleep, the body repairs and regenerates cells, including liver cells. Aim for 7-8 hours of uninterrupted sleep each night. Establish a relaxing bedtime routine, create a sleep-friendly environment, and prioritize good sleep hygiene practices.

Limit Exposure to Environmental Toxins:

Toxic substances in the environment can burden the liver and contribute to liver damage. Minimize exposure to environmental toxins by using natural and non-toxic cleaning products, avoiding excessive use of pesticides and insecticides, and being mindful of your surroundings. Additionally, consider investing in a high-quality water filter to reduce your exposure to contaminants in drinking water.

Conclusion:

Adopting lifestyle habits that support liver health is crucial for liver rejuvenation and overall well-being. By understanding the impact of alcohol, smoking, and stress on liver function, you can make informed decisions to minimize their negative effects. Embracing lifestyle changes such as following a balanced and nutritious diet, maintaining a healthy weight, staying hydrated, exercising regularly, getting sufficient sleep, and limiting exposure to environmental toxins can significantly contribute to liver rejuvenation.

Remember that every positive change you make in your lifestyle has a cumulative effect on your liver's health and function. It is important to approach these lifestyle changes as long-term commitments rather than short-term solutions. By prioritizing your liver's well-being and making conscious choices that support its rejuvenation, you are taking proactive steps toward a healthier and vibrant life. Consult with healthcare professionals or liver specialists for personalized advice and guidance tailored to your specific needs. Embrace these lifestyle habits, and let your liver thrive as you unlock your body's vitality.

Chapter 7: Exercise for Liver Health and Rejuvenation

Unveiling the relationship between physical activity and liver function

Designing an exercise routine that benefits liver health

Introduction:

Regular exercise is known to have numerous benefits for overall health, but its impact on liver health is often overlooked. Engaging in physical activity not only improves cardiovascular fitness, strengthens muscles, and enhances mental well-being but also plays a vital role in supporting liver function and rejuvenation. In this chapter, we will explore the relationship between exercise and liver health, as well as provide guidelines for designing an exercise routine that specifically benefits the liver.

The Relationship Between Physical Activity and Liver Function:

The liver is responsible for metabolizing nutrients, removing toxins, and maintaining metabolic homeostasis. Exercise has been shown to have a positive impact on liver health through various mechanisms. Here are some key ways in which physical activity benefits the liver:

1. Weight Management: Regular exercise helps maintain a healthy weight or achieve weight loss, which is crucial for liver health. Excess body weight, especially abdominal fat, increases the risk of non-alcoholic fatty liver disease (NAFLD) and other liver conditions. By engaging in exercise, you can reduce liver fat accumulation and improve liver function.

2. Insulin Sensitivity: Physical activity enhances insulin sensitivity, which is important for proper glucose metabolism and prevention of insulin resistance. Insulin resistance is closely linked to the development of NAFLD and type 2 diabetes. By improving insulin sensitivity through exercise, you can reduce the risk of liver-related complications.

3. Inflammation Reduction: Chronic inflammation is a key driver of liver damage and progression of liver diseases. Exercise has anti-inflammatory effects and helps reduce systemic inflammation, including liver inflammation. By decreasing inflammation, exercise promotes liver health and protects against liver damage.

4. Oxidative Stress Reduction: Oxidative stress occurs when there is an imbalance between free radicals and antioxidants in the body. Excessive oxidative stress can lead to liver cell damage. Regular exercise enhances the body's antioxidant defenses, reducing oxidative stress and supporting liver cell health.

5. Blood Flow Improvement: Exercise increases blood flow and oxygen delivery to various organs, including the liver. This enhanced blood flow improves nutrient

delivery and waste removal, supporting liver function and rejuvenation.

Designing an Exercise Routine for Liver Health:

To optimize liver health and rejuvenation, it is important to design an exercise routine that incorporates a variety of physical activities. Here are some guidelines to consider:

1. Aerobic Exercise: Engage in aerobic activities that increase heart rate and promote cardiovascular fitness. Examples include brisk walking, jogging, cycling, swimming, dancing, and aerobics classes. Aim for at least 150 minutes of moderate-intensity aerobic exercise or 75 minutes of vigorous-intensity aerobic exercise per week.

2. Strength Training: Include resistance exercises to build and maintain muscle strength. Strength training can be done using free weights, weight machines, resistance bands, or bodyweight exercises such as push-ups, squats, and lunges. Aim for two or more sessions per week, targeting major muscle groups.

3. Interval Training: Incorporate interval training into your routine. This involves alternating between high-intensity bursts of exercise and periods of lower intensity or rest. For example, alternate between sprinting and walking or cycling at a high intensity and then recovering at a lower intensity. Interval training can be effective for improving fitness, burning calories, and supporting liver health.

4. Flexibility and Balance Exercises: Include exercises that improve flexibility, such as stretching or yoga, and activities that enhance balance, such as tai chi or Pilates. These exercises help maintain joint mobility, improve posture, and reduce the risk of injuries during other physical activities.

5. Gradual Progression: Start with an exercise routine that matches your current fitness level and gradually progress over time. It is important to listen to your body and avoid over exertion. Gradually increase the duration, intensity, and frequency of your workouts as your fitness improves. Consulting with a healthcare professional or a certified fitness trainer can provide valuable guidance and help you create an exercise plan tailored to your individual needs and goals.

Additional Tips for Liver-Friendly Exercise:

1. Consistency is Key: Aim for regular exercise by incorporating physical activity into your daily routine. Consistency is important for reaping the long-term benefits of exercise for liver health. Find activities you enjoy and make them a priority.

2. Stay Hydrated: Drink plenty of water before, during, and after exercise to stay properly hydrated. Hydration supports optimal liver function and overall performance during physical activity.

3. Warm-Up and Cool Down: Always begin your exercise session with a warm-up to prepare your body for the workout and reduce the risk of injury.

Likewise, finish your exercise routine with a cool-down period to gradually lower your heart rate and allow your body to recover.

4. Listen to Your Body: Pay attention to any signs of discomfort or pain during exercise. If you experience persistent or severe symptoms, such as chest pain, shortness of breath, dizziness, or unusual fatigue, stop exercising and consult a healthcare professional.

5. Combine Exercise with a Healthy Lifestyle: Remember that exercise is just one piece of the puzzle for liver health. It should be complemented by a balanced diet, adequate sleep, stress management, and other healthy lifestyle habits.

Conclusion:

Exercise plays a crucial role in supporting liver health and rejuvenation. By engaging in regular physical activity, you can improve liver function, reduce the risk of liver diseases, and promote overall well-being. Physical activity helps manage weight, enhances insulin sensitivity, reduces inflammation and oxidative stress, and improves blood flow to the liver.

Designing an exercise routine that includes aerobic exercise, strength training, interval training, flexibility, and balance exercises can maximize the benefits for your liver. Remember to start at your current fitness level and gradually progress over time. Consistency, hydration, warm-up, and cool-down periods are important aspects of safe and effective exercise.

By incorporating exercise into your daily routine and making it a priority, you are taking proactive steps towards liver health. Combine exercise with a healthy lifestyle that includes a balanced diet, sufficient sleep, stress management, and other liver-friendly habits for comprehensive liver rejuvenation. Consult with healthcare professionals or fitness experts for personalized advice and guidance. Unlock the power of exercise to support your liver and experience the transformative effects on your overall health and vitality.

Chapter 8: Sleep and Liver Rejuvenation

The importance of quality sleep in liver rejuvenation

Tips for improving sleep habits to support liver health

Introduction:

Sleep is a fundamental aspect of our daily lives, and its importance extends beyond rest and relaxation. Quality sleep plays a crucial role in supporting overall health and well-being, including the rejuvenation of vital organs like the liver. In this chapter, we will explore the significance of sleep in liver rejuvenation and provide practical tips for improving sleep habits to support liver health.

The Importance of Quality Sleep in Liver Rejuvenation:

The liver performs essential functions in the body, including detoxification, metabolism, and nutrient storage. During sleep, the body undergoes a series of restorative processes that support liver health and rejuvenation. Here are some key reasons why quality sleep is vital for liver rejuvenation:

1. Detoxification: The liver works diligently to detoxify the body, removing harmful substances and waste products. During sleep, the brain's glymphatic system, a waste-clearing mechanism, becomes more active, allowing for the efficient removal of toxins

from the brain and other tissues, including the liver. Quality sleep supports optimal detoxification processes, allowing the liver to effectively perform its vital functions.

2. Cellular Repair and Regeneration: Sleep is a time of cellular repair and regeneration throughout the body, including the liver. During sleep, the liver can repair damaged cells and regenerate new healthy cells, optimizing its function and promoting overall liver health.

3. Regulation of Metabolic Processes: Sleep plays a crucial role in regulating various metabolic processes, including glucose metabolism. Sufficient sleep helps maintain balanced insulin levels and improves insulin sensitivity. By supporting healthy metabolic functioning, adequate sleep reduces the risk of developing conditions such as non-alcoholic fatty liver disease (NAFLD) and metabolic syndrome.

4. Inflammation Reduction: Chronic sleep deprivation can contribute to increased systemic inflammation, which is associated with liver damage and the progression of liver diseases. Quality sleep helps regulate inflammatory processes in the body, including the liver, reducing the risk of inflammation-related liver conditions.

Tips for Improving Sleep Habits to Support Liver Health:

To optimize sleep quality and support liver rejuvenation, it is important to establish healthy sleep habits. Here are some practical tips to improve your sleep routine:

1. Stick to a Consistent Sleep Schedule: Aim to go to bed and wake up at the same time each day, including weekends. Consistency helps regulate your body's internal clock and promotes better sleep quality.

2. Create a Relaxing Bedtime Routine: Develop a pre-sleep routine that signals to your body that it's time to wind down and prepare for sleep. This may include activities such as reading a book, taking a warm bath, practicing relaxation techniques, or listening to calming music. Avoid stimulating activities or electronics close to bedtime, as they can interfere with sleep quality.

3. Create a Sleep-Friendly Environment: Ensure that your sleep environment is conducive to quality sleep. Keep your bedroom cool, quiet, and dark. Use curtains, blinds, or an eye mask to block out excess light. Consider using white noise machines or earplugs to mask any disturbing sounds.

4. Limit Exposure to Electronic Devices: The blue light emitted by electronic devices such as smartphones, tablets, and computers can disrupt your sleep-wake cycle. Avoid using these devices for at least an hour before bed or use blue light filters or apps that reduce blue light emissions.

5. Avoid Stimulants: Limit your intake of stimulants such as caffeine and nicotine, especially in the hours leading up to bedtime. These substances can

interfere with sleep quality and make it more difficult to fall asleep.

6. Engage in Regular Physical Activity: Regular exercise during the day can promote better sleep at night. However, avoid exercising too close to bedtime, as it can be stimulating and make it harder to fall asleep. Aim to finish your exercise routine at least a few hours before bed to allow your body to wind down.

7. Manage Stress: Stress can significantly impact sleep quality. Find healthy ways to manage stress, such as practicing relaxation techniques (e.g., deep breathing, meditation, yoga) or engaging in activities that help you unwind and clear your mind. Prioritize self-care and make time for activities that bring you joy and relaxation.

8. Create a Comfortable Sleep Environment: Invest in a comfortable mattress, pillows, and bedding that suit your preferences. Ensure your bedroom is well-ventilated and the temperature is cool and comfortable for sleep. If necessary, use sleep aids such as blackout curtains, earplugs, or white noise machines to create a serene sleeping environment.

9. Limit Fluid Intake Before Bed: Minimize your consumption of fluids, especially caffeine and alcohol, in the evening. This can help reduce the frequency of nighttime awakenings due to bathroom visits and promote uninterrupted sleep.

10. Seek Professional Help if Needed: If you consistently struggle with poor sleep quality or have symptoms of a sleep disorder such as insomnia or sleep apnea, it is advisable to seek professional help. A sleep specialist can provide a comprehensive evaluation, diagnosis, and appropriate treatment options tailored to your specific needs.

Conclusion:

Quality sleep is a vital component of liver rejuvenation and overall health. By prioritizing and improving your sleep habits, you can support the optimal functioning and rejuvenation of your liver. Adequate sleep promotes detoxification, cellular repair and regeneration, regulation of metabolic processes, and reduction of inflammation, all of which contribute to liver health.

Incorporate the tips mentioned in this chapter into your daily routine to establish healthy sleep habits. Consistency, a relaxing bedtime routine, a sleep-friendly environment, limiting electronic device use, managing stress, regular physical activity, and seeking professional help when needed are key factors in improving sleep quality and supporting liver rejuvenation.

Remember that sleep is a fundamental pillar of health and making sleep a priority can have far-reaching benefits beyond liver health. Embrace the power of quality sleep to unlock your body's vitality and optimize your overall well-being.

Special Report:

If you check any of these boxes:

- Have a hard time falling asleep.
- Can get to sleep, but you can't stay asleep.
- Wake up with a million things racing through your mind—at 2 AM.
- Have mood swings that range from overly happy to downright angry.
- You always have something "on the tip of your tongue," but can't remember what it is.
- Often feel lost, out-of-sorts, or just confused.
- Are grumpy the minute you wake up.

Then it's clear you're suffering from sleep deprivation—and you need to fix it fast.

Here is a special report that I have created called "The Ultimate Sleep Guide".

www.JayLabPro.com/Ultimate-Sleep-Guide.html

Chapter 9: Mind-Body Connection: Mental Wellness for Liver Rejuvenation

Exploring the link between emotional well-being and liver health

Strategies for managing stress, anxiety, and promoting mental wellness

Introduction:

The connection between our mental and physical well-being is undeniable. Our emotions, thoughts, and stress levels can impact various aspects of our health, including the well-being of our vital organs such as the liver. In this chapter, we will delve into the link between emotional well-being and liver health, and provide strategies for managing stress, anxiety, and promoting mental wellness to support liver rejuvenation.

The Link Between Emotional Well-being and Liver Health:

The liver, a resilient organ responsible for detoxification, metabolism, and storage of nutrients, is influenced by our mental and emotional state. Here are some key ways in which emotional well-being can impact liver health:

1. Stress and Cortisol: Chronic stress triggers the release of cortisol, a hormone that, in excess, can lead to inflammation and damage in the liver.

Prolonged exposure to stress can disrupt liver function and contribute to the development or progression of liver diseases.

2. Emotional Eating and Unhealthy Habits: Emotional factors, such as stress, anxiety, and depression, can influence our eating behaviors. Emotional eating, often characterized by the consumption of unhealthy, high-fat, or sugary foods, can contribute to weight gain, liver fat accumulation, and the development of liver conditions such as non-alcoholic fatty liver disease (NAFLD).

3. Inflammation and Immune Function: Emotional stress and negative emotions can trigger inflammation in the body, including the liver. Chronic inflammation can impair liver function and contribute to the progression of liver diseases. Additionally, stress can weaken the immune system, making the liver more susceptible to infections and impairing its ability to heal and rejuvenate.

Strategies for Managing Stress, Anxiety, and Promoting Mental Wellness:

To support liver rejuvenation and overall health, it is essential to prioritize mental wellness and adopt strategies to manage stress and anxiety. Here are some effective strategies:

1. Mindfulness and Meditation: Practicing mindfulness and meditation techniques can help reduce stress, promote relaxation, and improve emotional well-being. Engaging in regular

mindfulness exercises, such as deep breathing, body scans, or guided meditation, can help cultivate a sense of calm and balance.

2. Exercise and Physical Activity: Regular exercise not only benefits physical health but also plays a crucial role in promoting mental well-being. Physical activity releases endorphins, the "feel-good" hormones, which can alleviate stress, boost mood, and enhance overall mental wellness. Incorporate activities you enjoy, such as walking, yoga, dancing, or any form of exercise that brings you joy.

3. Social Support: Cultivate a strong support network of family, friends, or support groups. Sharing your feelings and experiences with trusted individuals can provide emotional support, reduce feelings of isolation, and contribute to improved mental well-being. Connecting with others who understand and empathize with your journey can be immensely helpful.

4. Cognitive-Behavioral Techniques: Cognitive-behavioral techniques, such as cognitive restructuring and reframing, can help manage stress, anxiety, and negative thinking patterns. Engaging in self-reflection, challenging negative thoughts, and adopting positive affirmations can promote mental wellness and resilience.

5. Healthy Coping Mechanisms: Identify healthy coping mechanisms that work for you, such as engaging in hobbies, practicing relaxation techniques, journaling, or seeking professional therapy or

counseling. Developing healthy ways to cope with stress and manage emotions can significantly contribute to mental well-being.

6. Self-Care Practices: Prioritize self-care activities that nourish your mind, body, and soul. This may include activities such as getting sufficient sleep, engaging in self-care practices, maintaining a healthy diet, engaging in hobbies and activities you enjoy, spending time in nature, practicing gratitude, and setting boundaries to protect your mental well-being. Taking time for yourself and engaging in activities that bring you joy and relaxation can help alleviate stress and promote a positive mindset.

7. Stress Reduction Techniques: Explore different stress reduction techniques to find what works best for you. This may include practices such as deep breathing exercises, progressive muscle relaxation, aromatherapy, or engaging in activities that promote relaxation, such as taking baths or practicing yoga. Find activities that help you unwind and reduce stress levels.

8. Seek Professional Support: If you are experiencing persistent stress, anxiety, or other mental health concerns, it is important to seek professional help. A mental health professional can provide guidance, support, and evidence-based therapies to address your specific needs. Therapy, counseling, or other modalities can be instrumental in managing stress, anxiety, and promoting mental wellness.

9. Practice Gratitude and Positive Thinking: Cultivate a mindset of gratitude and focus on the positive aspects of your life. Keeping a gratitude journal, expressing appreciation for the things you have, and reframing negative thoughts into more positive ones can shift your perspective and promote emotional well-being.

10. Balance Work and Leisure: Strive for a healthy work-life balance by setting boundaries and making time for leisure activities. Engage in hobbies, spend quality time with loved ones, and allow yourself periods of relaxation and enjoyment. Prioritizing leisure and downtime is essential for mental rejuvenation and overall well-being.

Conclusion:

The mind-body connection is a powerful aspect of our well-being, and nurturing our mental health is crucial for liver rejuvenation. By understanding the link between emotional well-being and liver health, and adopting strategies to manage stress, anxiety, and promote mental wellness, we can support the optimal functioning of our liver and enhance overall health.

Incorporate mindfulness and meditation practices, engage in regular exercise, seek social support, practice healthy coping mechanisms, prioritize self-care, and explore stress reduction techniques to manage stress and promote emotional well-being. Remember to seek professional support when needed, as trained professionals can provide valuable guidance and support tailored to your individual needs.

By prioritizing mental wellness and implementing strategies to manage stress and anxiety, you are taking proactive steps to support liver rejuvenation and enhance your overall quality of life. Embrace the mind-body connection, nurture your emotional well-being, and unlock the transformative power of mental wellness in your journey towards optimal liver health.

Chapter 10: Long-Term Liver Rejuvenation: Maintenance and Prevention

Maintaining a healthy liver beyond rejuvenation

Preventive measures to ensure long-term liver health and vitality

Introduction:

Liver rejuvenation is a transformative process that restores the health and vitality of one of the body's most important organs. However, it is equally important to focus on long-term maintenance and prevention to ensure ongoing liver health. In this final chapter, we will explore strategies for maintaining a healthy liver beyond rejuvenation and implementing preventive measures to safeguard long-term liver health and vitality.

Maintaining a Healthy Liver Beyond Rejuvenation:

After successfully rejuvenating the liver, it is crucial to maintain its health and functionality. Here are some key strategies to consider:

1. Continued Healthy Diet: Maintain a well-balanced and nutritious diet that supports liver health. Emphasize whole foods, including fruits, vegetables, whole grains, lean proteins, and healthy fats. Limit the consumption of processed foods, sugary

beverages, and foods high in saturated and trans fats. Be mindful of portion sizes and practice moderation.

2. Regular Exercise: Continue engaging in regular physical activity to support liver health and overall well-being. Aim for a combination of cardiovascular exercise, strength training, and flexibility exercises. Regular exercise helps maintain a healthy weight, improves insulin sensitivity, and promotes optimal liver function.

3. Moderate Alcohol Consumption: If you choose to consume alcohol, do so in moderation. Excessive alcohol consumption can damage the liver and lead to conditions such as alcoholic liver disease. Follow the recommended guidelines for moderate alcohol intake, which vary depending on gender and individual circumstances.

4. Avoid Hepatotoxic Substances: Be cautious of substances that can be harmful to the liver. This includes certain medications, herbal supplements, and recreational drugs. Consult with healthcare professionals before taking any medications or supplements, especially if you have a pre-existing liver condition.

5. Regular Liver Check-ups: Schedule regular check-ups with your healthcare provider to monitor your liver health. They can perform liver function tests, assess your overall health, and provide guidance on maintaining optimal liver function. Regular check-ups enable early detection of any potential issues and allow for prompt intervention if needed.

6. Maintain a Healthy Weight: Strive to maintain a healthy weight through a combination of a balanced diet and regular exercise. Obesity and excess body weight can contribute to liver fat accumulation and increase the risk of conditions such as non-alcoholic fatty liver disease (NAFLD). Aim for gradual, sustainable weight loss if necessary.

7. Manage Chronic Conditions: If you have any chronic conditions, such as diabetes, high blood pressure, or high cholesterol, work closely with your healthcare team to manage and control these conditions effectively. Uncontrolled chronic conditions can have a negative impact on liver health.

8. Stay Hydrated: Drink an adequate amount of water daily to support optimal liver function. Water helps flush out toxins and waste products from the body, aiding in liver detoxification processes. Aim to drink at least 8 glasses of water per day, or more if you are physically active or live in a hot climate.

Preventive Measures for Long-Term Liver Health and Vitality:

In addition to maintaining a healthy liver, implementing preventive measures is essential to ensure long-term liver health and vitality. Here are some important preventive measures to consider:

1. Vaccinations: Protect yourself against viral infections that can affect the liver, such as hepatitis A and B. Ensure you are up-to-date with recommended

vaccinations and follow any additional recommendations provided by healthcare professionals.

2. Practice Safe Sex: Engage in safe sexual practices to prevent the transmission of sexually transmitted infections (STIs) that can affect liver health. Use barrier methods of contraception, such as condoms, and limit sexual partners.

3. Practice Good Hygiene: Practice good hygiene habits to reduce the risk of infections that can impact liver health. This includes regular handwashing with soap and water, especially before handling food or after using the restroom. Avoid sharing personal hygiene items, such as toothbrushes or razors, to minimize the risk of infection transmission.

4. Maintain a Healthy Gut: The health of your gut microbiome can influence liver health. Consume a diet rich in fiber to support a healthy gut microbiome and promote regular bowel movements. Probiotic-rich foods, such as yogurt and fermented foods, can also help maintain a healthy balance of gut bacteria.

5. Avoid Environmental Toxins: Minimize exposure to environmental toxins and chemicals that can be harmful to the liver. This includes reducing exposure to pesticides, cleaning chemicals, and other toxic substances. Use protective gear, such as gloves and masks, when handling potentially hazardous materials.

6. Practice Safe Medication Use: Follow proper medication practices to prevent adverse effects on the liver. Take medications as prescribed, avoid self-medication, and inform healthcare providers about any existing liver conditions or concerns. Be aware of potential interactions between medications and herbal supplements.

7. Limit Exposure to Hepatitis-Causing Risk Factors: Hepatitis C is a viral infection that can lead to liver damage. Limit exposure to risk factors such as intravenous drug use, unsafe tattoo or piercing practices, and unprotected sex with multiple partners. If you suspect exposure to hepatitis C, seek medical attention for testing and appropriate treatment.

8. Stress Management: Chronic stress can impact liver health. Implement stress management techniques such as relaxation exercises, meditation, mindfulness, and engaging in activities that promote relaxation and emotional well-being. Seek support from mental health professionals if needed.

9. Educate Yourself: Stay informed about liver health and the latest research and recommendations. Educate yourself about liver diseases, risk factors, and prevention strategies. Being knowledgeable empowers you to make informed decisions and take proactive steps to protect your liver.

10. Foster a Supportive Lifestyle: Surround yourself with a supportive network of family and friends who encourage and support your commitment to liver

health. Share your journey with them, seek their understanding, and engage in activities that promote a healthy lifestyle together.

Conclusion:

Maintaining a healthy liver beyond the rejuvenation process requires ongoing dedication and preventive measures. By following a healthy lifestyle, practicing moderation, staying informed, and seeking regular medical check-ups, you can ensure long-term liver health and vitality.

Remember that the liver is a remarkable organ with incredible regenerative abilities. By implementing the strategies outlined in this book and adopting a proactive approach to liver health, you can enjoy the benefits of a healthy liver for years to come. Embrace the power of maintenance and prevention and make liver health a priority in your journey towards optimal well-being.

Appendix A

Liver Rejuvenation 7-Day Sample Meal Plan

Day 1:

Breakfast:
1 Egg (Cooked any style or hard-boiled)
1 Apple with Tahini butter
Cut Vegetables (could be mixed with egg)
Unsweetened Cranberry Drink

Midmorning Snack:
1/3 cup nuts or seeds

Lunch
Salad (almonds, kales, collard greens, broccoli sprouts, carrots)
Drizzle balsamic vinegar and olive oil over it.
1 serving of fruit
3 oz. chicken breast.

Afternoon Snack:
1 apple
½ cup plain Greek yogurt

Dinner:
3-4oz Fish
Lentils
Mixed Vegetables
Avocado
Unsweetened Cranberry Drink

Evening Snack:
½ cup of fruit
½ cup of nuts

Day 2:

Breakfast:
½ cup cottage cheese
½ cup of berries
¼ cup walnuts
Unsweetened Cranberry Drink

Morning Snack:
Mixed Vegetables
Hard-boiled egg

Lunch:
3-4 oz Fish
A variety of vegetables
Apple

Afternoon Snack:
¼ cup seeds or nuts
½ cup plain Greek yogurt
Dinner:
3-4oz Salmon
Lentils
Vegetables
½ cup fruit
Unsweetened Cranberry drink

Evening Snack:

½ cup plain Greek yogurt
Apple
Day 3:

Breakfast:
1 egg
½ cup berries
Vegetables mixed with egg
A small amount of cheese to top egg with
Unsweetened Cranberry Drink

Morning snack:
Vegetables
½ cup of pistachios

Lunch:
3-4 oz Tuna over a bed of greens/salad with a variety
of vegetables
Apple
Seeds to top Salad with
Afternoon Snack:
½ cup cottage cheese
½ cup fruit
¼ cup walnuts

Dinner:
3-4oz Turkey
Vegetables (could make into a salad with chicken or
turkey)
Lentils
Apple
Unsweetened Cranberry Juice

Evening Snack:
Hard-boiled egg
Raw vegetables

Day 4:

Breakfast:
Greek yogurt with raspberries and almonds
Hard-boiled egg
½ avocado sliced drizzled with extra virgin olive oil
and lemon juice

Morning snack:
Apple
Pistachios
Lunch:
Mixed greens salad with sliced beets, walnuts,
mozzarella cheese
4oz sliced chicken
Finish with a balsamic vinaigrette dressing

Afternoon Snack:
Sliced cucumbers
Carrot Sticks
Guacamole (use as a dip for the vegetables)

Dinner:
4 oz. Fish
Variety of mixed vegetables. (preferably raw, but
lightly steamed works also)
Pine Nuts

Evening Snack:
Apple
Cottage Cheese

Day 5:

Breakfast:
Scrambled Eggs (mixed with mushrooms, green peppers, onion, spinach)
Sprinkled with cheese
Unsweetened Cranberry Drink
Morning snack:
Apple
Greek yogurt with walnuts

Lunch:
Tuna Salad on lettuce leaves
Roasted brussels sprouts

Afternoon Snack:
Brie cheese with sliced pears

Dinner:
Spaghetti squash tossed with fresh herbs and olive oil
Diced hard-boiled egg (mix with spaghetti squash)
Hummus with celery sticks

Evening Snack:
Cottage Cheese
Blueberries

Day 6:

Breakfast:
Sliced Apples with Peanut Butter
Walnuts
Sliced Vegetables

Morning snack:
Greek yogurt with chopped pecans

Lunch:
Baby Spinach Salad with
Broccoli sprouts
Celery
Carrots
Kale
Avocado
Sugar snap peas
4 oz. Fish or Tuna Salad

Afternoon Snack:
Apple
Cottage Cheese

Dinner:
4oz chicken
diced tomato
broccoli sprouts
avocado slices
brie cheese
Bibb Lettuce leaves (wrap above ingredients into
lettuce leaves)

Evening Snack:
Pistachios
Celery Sticks and Peanut Butter

Day 7:

Breakfast:
Hard-Boiled Egg
Cottage Cheese with Peaches
Unsweetened Cranberry Drink

Morning snack:
Grapefruit
Hard-Boiled Egg

Lunch:
Tuna Salad
Cauliflower sautéed in coconut oil

Afternoon Snack:
Apple with Tahini
Sliced vegetables

Dinner:
Apple Turkey Burger (no bun)
Mushrooms sautéed in butter
Sautéed Brussel sprouts, asparagus, sugar snap peas, carrots, sunflower seeds

Evening Snack:
String Cheese
Celery with Peanut Butter

Appendix B

Recipes

Tuna Salad

Two 6-ounce can of white albacore tuna packed in oil, drained
2 Tbsp. celery, minced
2 Tbsp. red onion, minced
1 tsp minced parsley
1/3 cup Greek yogurt
1 Tbsp. Dijon mustard
2 Tbsp. sweet pickle relish
Freshly squeezed lemon juice

Directions:

In a small bowl break up the tuna with a fork. Toss in the celery, onion, and parsley. Add the Greek yogurt, mustard, pickle relish, add lemon juice to taste

Spaghetti Squash

1 medium spaghetti squash, halved lengthwise and seeded.
¼ cup extra virgin olive oil
4 cloves garlic, minced
½ cup pecans, toasted
¼ cup grated Asiago cheese
1.5 tsps. fresh lemon juice
½ bunch of parsley

Directions:

Preheat the oven to 375 degrees. Rub the cut sides of the squash with 1 tsp of olive oil and sprinkle with salt and pepper. Set them on a baking sheet with the cut side down. Place the cloves of garlic on a piece of foil and drizzle with the olive oil.

Wrap up the foil to form a pouch and place it onto the baking sheet with the squash. Bake until the squash is tender and the garlic is roasted. It should take about 35-40 minutes.

Once the garlic cloves have cooled place them into a food processor along with the toasted pecans, parsley, and ½ tsp salt. Once pulverized drizzle in ½ cup extra virgin olive oil. Then add the shredded asiago cheese and lemon juice. Only blend until combined.

Shred the squash into a bowl using a fork and mix with the pesto you just made.

Ginger Kale Salad

2-3 cups Kale and chopped into 2-inch pieces
2 Tbsp. sesame seeds
1 Tbsp. ginger, minced
2 Tbsp. toasted sesame oil
2 Tbsp. apple cider vinegar
1/8 tsp coarse ground pepper
1/8 tsp sea salt

Directions:

In a large bowl, place the kale, and then in another
small bowl mix together the ginger, sesame oil, apple
cider vinegar, salt, and pepper. Whisk together well
and then drizzle over kale. Top with sesame seeds
and enjoy!

Roasted Cauliflower, Onions, Sweet Potatoes

3 cups fresh cauliflower florets
6 ounces' sweet potato, peeled and cut into ¾ inch
cubes
1 medium onion, cut into wedges
¼ tsp nutmeg
¼ tsp turmeric

Directions:

Preheat oven to 425 degrees. On a large foiled
baking sheet place the cauliflower, sweet potatoes,
and onion. Drizzle the vegetables with oil and gently
toss until they are well coated.

Once coated spread the vegetables out in a single
layer and bake for 10 minutes. Remove from oven
and stir. Then place back in the oven for another 10
minutes or until potatoes are tender.

Serve and enjoy!

Strawberry Pear Salad and White Balsamic Dressing

4 cups spinach
½ a pear, sliced thinly
1.5 cups strawberries. Sliced or quartered
½ cup red onion, thinly sliced

Dressing:

1/3 cup white balsamic vinegar
2.5 Tbsp. extra virgin olive oil
¼ tsp sea salt
¼ tsp coarsely ground black pepper
1/8 tsp dried red pepper flakes
1 ounce crumbled feta or blue cheese

Directions:

In a small bowl, whisk together the ingredients for
the dressing and spoon over the salad.

This makes 4 cups of salad so if you are not going to
eat all of it in one sitting then save some of the
dressing to use later with the rest of the salad.

Egg & Avocado Sandwich

1 egg (could be scrambled or fried)
4 tsp extra virgin olive oil
1 Tbsp. shredded mozzarella cheese
2 slices of avocado
Sweet potato sliced thinly (This will be your
toast/bread)

Directions:

Take 2 thin slices of sweet potato and put them into your toaster. Set the setting to high and you may have to toast them for 2-4 cycles for them to brown and toast up.

In a small frying pan add your olive oil and heat the pan. When the oil is hot crack your egg, and add it to the frying pan. Cook for 3 minutes or until the whites turn opaque.

Place one slice of toasted sweet potato on your plates and top it with your egg. Add your sprinkled cheese and then 2 slices of avocado. Finally, add your last slice of sweet potato toast and enjoy.

Turkey, Cranberry Spinach and Kale Salad

1.5 cups spinach
1.5 cups kale
1 cup cooked turkey breast, chopped into small chunks
2 stalks celery, diced
2-4 scallions, chopped
¾ cup cranberries, chopped
¼ cup balsamic vinaigrette dressing
½ cup pecan, chopped

Directions:

Place the spinach and kale spread out on a plate. Top the salad with the turkey, celery, scallions, and cranberries. Then drizzle the vinaigrette dressing over the salad. Finally, top with the chopped pecans and enjoy.

Black Rice Fruit Salad

¾ cup black rice
1 mango, cubed
2 cups strawberries, quartered
2 apples, chopped
1/3 cup cashews
Juice and zest of 1 lime
2 cups plain Greek yogurt
1 Tbsp. honey

Directions: Place rice and 1.5 cups of water into a saucepan. Bring to a boil and then reduce the heat to a simmer and cover for 25 minutes or until rice is tender and water has been absorbed. Set aside and keep covered for 5 minutes and then fluff with a fork.

In a large bowl mix the mango, strawberries, apples, cashews, and lime juice. In a separate bowl mix, together with the lime zest, yogurt, and honey.
Top the salad with the yogurt mixture and enjoy!

Butternut Hummus
1 pound butternut squash, peeled and diced
3 Tbsp. extra virgin olive oil
1 cup cooked chickpeas, drained and rinsed
1 garlic clove, minced
Juice from ½ a lemon
2 Tbsp. Tahini
1 tsp smoked paprika
½ tsp sea salt
½ tsp cumin powder
¼ tsp cinnamon
½ tsp turmeric

Directions:

Preheat oven to 400 degrees. Place the diced butternut squash with 1 tsp olive oil spread out on a baking sheet. Roast until tender or about 30 minutes. Remove from oven and let cool.

Once cooled place the butternut squash and remaining ingredients in a food processor or blender until blended smooth.

Caramelized Brussels Sprouts

This recipe serves 3 at 1 cup per serving.
2 Tbsp. extra virgin olive oil
½ yellow onion, chopped finely
1 pound Brussels sprouts, chopped
½ tsp minced garlic
2 tsp balsamic vinegar
1/8 tsp sea salt
1/8 tsp coarse ground black pepper

Directions:

Heat the olive oil in a skillet over medium heat. Add the onions, Brussel sprouts, and garlic. Sauté them for about 10 minutes while occasionally stirring the mixture until the Brussel sprouts are tender and browned.

Add the vinegar, sea salt, and pepper and continue to cook for about 5 more minutes. You may need to turn down the heat if the Brussel sprouts start to become too brown.

Spinach and Orange Salad with Pumpkin Seeds

1 cup spinach leaves
2 tsp diced celery
2 small mushrooms, sliced
1 red onion thinly sliced
½ medium orange, peeled and sectioned
2 Tbsp. fresh-squeezed orange juice
1 Tbsp. fresh lemon juice
1 Tbsp. extra virgin olive oil
1 tsp soy sauce
1 tsp honey
1/8 tsp ground ginger
1/8 tsp ground turmeric
1 Tbsp. roasted pumpkin seeds.

Directions:

In a medium bowl mix the spinach leaves, celery, mushrooms, onion, and orange sections. In a separate bowl whisk, together with the liquid ingredients. Once mixed drizzle over the salad and then top with the pumpkin seeds.

Cucumber Salad

Besides serving plain slices of cucumber on a lettuce leaf, as may be done at any time, cucumbers may be used as an ingredient in the making of many salads.

1   medium-sized cucumbers
1 c. diced tomato
1/2 c. diced celery
Balsamic Vinaigrette salad dressing
Lettuce
1 pimiento

Directions:

Peel the cucumbers cut them into halves, and with a small spoon scoop out the cucumbers in chunks so that a boat-shaped piece of cucumber that is about 1/4-inch-thick remains. Dice the pieces of cucumber which have been scooped from the center, and place the cucumber shells in ice water to make them crisp. Mix the diced tomato, celery, and cucumber, and just before serving drain them carefully so that no liquid remains. Mix with salad dressing, wipe the cucumber shells dry, fill them with the salad mixture, and place on salad plates garnished with lettuce leaves. Cut the pimiento into thin strips, and place three or four strips diagonally across the cucumber.

CARROT AND CABBAGE SALAD

1 medium-sized carrot
2 cups cabbage
1/2 cup walnuts
Italian Dressing

Directions:

Clean and scrape the carrot. Wash the cabbage. Put the carrot (uncooked), cabbage, and walnuts in a food processor. Mix with Italian Salad Dressing. Add more seasoning if necessary.

Egg Salad

6 hard-boiled eggs, chilled and peeled
¼ cup Greek yogurt
½ tsp lemon zest
1.5 tsps. fresh lemon juice
1/3 cup celery, diced
¼ cup scallions, chopped
1 Tbsp. fresh parsley, minced
Salt and pepper to taste

Directions:

In a small bowl break up the eggs into small chunks and then combine the yogurt, lemon juice, celery, scallions, and parsley. Mix with a fork or whisk until it reaches the consistency that you desire.

Serve in a lettuce wrap or use as a dip with celery.

Apple Mushroom Turkey Burgers

1lb ground turkey breast
5 mushrooms, finely chopped
1/2 small onion, finely chopped
1/2 apple, finely chopped
1/2 tablespoon coconut oil
1tsp lemon juice
1 omega---3 egg
1/2 tsp salt
garlic powder and pepper to taste

Directions:

Fry onion until brown. Then add the apples and mushrooms and stir---fry for another 4 minutes. Place all the ingredients into a large bowl and mix thoroughly. Form into 2 large patties and broil 4 inches from heat, 6 minutes on each side. The burgers are done when the juice runs clear after being pierced with a fork.

Farmer's Market Squash Sauté

2 yellow squash, sliced
2 zucchinis, sliced
2 cloves garlic, minced
1 Tbsp. extra virgin olive oil
½ cup 2% Mozzarella cheese
2 Tbsp. Chopped basil
2 Tbsp. Grated Parmesan cheese

Directions:

Cook Zucchini and squash in hot oil in a large skillet on medium heat for 3 min. stirring occasionally. Add garlic; cook 3 min. or until vegetables are crisp---tender. Remove from heat; stir in mozzarella and basil. Sprinkle with Parmesan.

Orange Tangy Barbecue Chicken with Vegetables

1/4 cup Barbecue Sauce (see recipe below)
1/4 tsp. grated orange peel
1 Tbsp. fresh orange juice
2 boneless skinless chicken breast halves (about 1/2 lb.)
1 small zucchini, cut lengthwise in half
1 small yellow squash, cut lengthwise in half
1 medium red pepper, cut into quarters
2 Tbsp. Light Italian Dressing

Directions:

Preheat grill to medium heat. Mix barbecue sauce, orange peel, and juice until well blended; set aside. Grill chicken for 6 min., turning over after 3 min. Brush with barbecue sauce mixture. Add vegetables to the grill. Continue grilling chicken and vegetables for 9 to 12 min. or until chicken is cooked through (170ºF) and vegetables are tender, turning occasionally and brushing chicken with the remaining barbecue sauce mixture and vegetables with the dressing.

Tangy Barbecue Sauce

4 cups sliced strawberries
1/2 cup chili sauce
2 Tbsp. apple cider vinegar
2 Tbsp. Worcestershire sauce
1/2 tsp lemon zest
2 Tbsp. fresh lemon juice
1 large garlic clove, minced
1 Tbsp. light brown sugar
1/2 tsp sea salt
1/2 tsp cayenne pepper

Directions:

In a food processor mix all the ingredients until smooth.

Italian Dressing Recipe

1 cup apple cider vinegar
1 1/4 cup extra virgin olive oil
1 tbsp. garlic powder
1 tbsp. onion powder
1 tbsp. Italian herb
1 tsp. Dijon mustard, no sugar added
1 tsp. dried basil
1/2 tsp. ground black pepper
1/4 tsp. sea salt

Directions:

Combine the ingredients in a blender and blend
well.

Tangy Broccoli Salad

3/4 cup Greek yogurt
2 Tbsp. sugar
2 Tbsp. vinegar
1 bunch broccoli, cut into florets (6 cups)
6 slices Turkey Bacon, crisply cooked, drained, and
crumbled
1 small red onion, chopped

Directions:

Mix dressing, sugar, and vinegar in a large bowl.
Add remaining ingredients; mix lightly.
Refrigerate at least 1 hour before serving.

Guacamole

2 ripe avocados
1/2 tsp sea salt
1 Tbsp. of fresh lime juice or lemon juice
3 Tbsp. minced red onion
1-2 serrano chills, stems and seeds removed, minced
2 tablespoons cilantro (leaves and tender stems),
finely chopped

A dash of freshly grated black pepper
1/2 ripe tomato, seeds and pulp removed, chopped

Directions:

Cut the avocado in half and remove the seed. Then
scoop out the flesh. Mash with a fork, but leave it a
little chunky.   Add salt, lime juice, and the remaining
ingredients.   If this will be something that you will
keep on hand to snack on I would leave the tomatoes
out of the recipe and only add them right before
eating it.

Resources:

https://www.jaylabpro.com/What-Your-Doctor-NEVER-Told-You-About-Fish-Oil.html

https://www.jaylabpro.com/14-Foods-Heal-Liver.html

https://www.jaylabpro.com/7-Foods-That-Fight-Inflammation.html

https://www.jaylabpro.com/5-Blood-Tests.html

https://www.jaylabpro.com/15-worst-hidden-sugar-foods.html

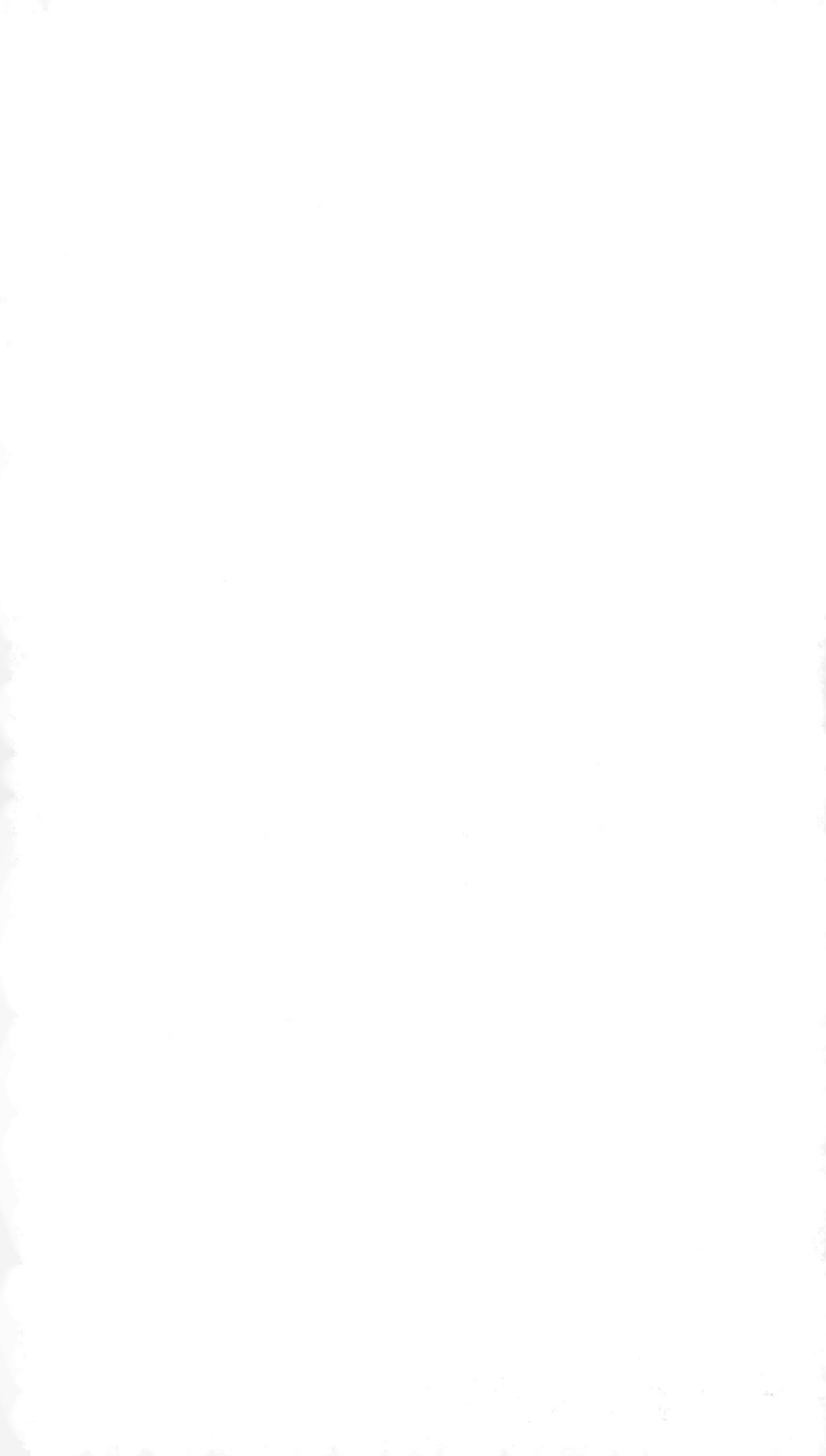

www.ingramcontent.com/pod-product-compliance
Lightning Source LLC
Chambersburg PA
CBHW060953260726
48661CB00005B/1873